Table of Contents

Introduction

First I would like to thank and congratulate you for investing in

Emotional Intelligence The Secrets To Developing The Star Potential In Your Child.

Within the pages of these books you will be given suggestions on quick methods that will help you raise your child's emotional intelligence, how you can apply these methods, as well as what to do if you run into a roadblock along the way. By using the tips and suggestions offered in this book you are going to improve and enrich the life of your child by empowering their skills that will lead to them being able to manage and work with their emotions instead of against them.

There tend to be conflicting ideas when it comes to emotional intelligence, some are of the opinion that this is a natural ability that no amount of training or practice will effect it. Others believe that it is a measurement of the person's current ability, which is built upon a mix of natural talent, instruction and practice.

What I will be referencing here within the pages of this book will be an emotional intelligence that is a complex interaction between inborn skills, and instruction and experience.

Using a process of social-emotional learning blended with the person's natural personality traits, and preferences; it is possible to teach the skills and attitudes that are necessary to improve a person's emotional intelligence. Of course the type of personal traits that you are dealing with can have a large impact on the results. At least as a parent or even as a teacher you will have a more intimate understanding of themselves and their child or student. The personal qualities will certainly have a huge impact on the total learning process. You will find that methods that can work great for one child may not work at all for another child. Even siblings are going to develop and learn differently. But just keep in mind that it is possible to raise your child's emotional intelligence through instruction, and it is also a very important and vital part of their overall well-being.

Chapter 1

Overview and Understanding of Emotional Intelligence

Emotional Intelligence or "EI" is one of the many types of intelligence that is now accepted in general psychology today. Howard Gardner (Professor of Cognition and Education at the Harvard Graduate School of Education at Harvard University) originally had intelligence split into nine different categories. In his setup he has explained that humans have different skills and abilities, different "intelligence," that relate to different areas or things. For example, we have some people that have what we refer to as "word smart" having the natural ability to use language either written or spoken. There are people that have the "body smarts" that have natural good coordination and predilection for athletics. An offshoot term of the multiple intelligence theory. This is not one of the original ones that Gardner had coined, but it still fits well within these.

The common description for emotional intelligence is defined as a person having the ability to be able to reason with emotions and to use them in enhancing their thought patterns.

A person that possesses high emotional intelligence can do the following:

quickly identify emotions in themselves as well as others

make use of those emotions in order to facilitate thoughts and actions

are able to understand what emotions mean and can analyze what could be causing them

able to manage and control their own emotions

The four basic branches of emotional intelligence coincide with the skills mentioned above. Each of these branches is interrelated and individuals. It is possible for a person to be weaker in one branch compared to another. All of the branches come together to complete an overall picture of the person's emotional intelligence.

Understanding Emotions

If a child is able to understand and recognize an emotion as "angry" or "happy", but is unable to know that it means, then they will not be able to

take the appropriate action. Being able to understand is the ability to be able
to recognize the social information that is being conveyed through the use of
emotions.

Perceiving Emotion

This is usually what we are referring to when we are talking about a person that has empathy and high sympathy for others. They are able to understand how that person is feeling based on non-verbal cues. They do not need to be verbally told that the person is feeling hurt, angry or upset in some way.

Using Emotions to Facilitate Thought

When a person realizes that an emotion exists they must then allow their thoughts to guide them towards the appropriate form of action. This can readily be seen in children, as they are developing their emotional intelligence there is usually noticeable gaps. A child, for example, may see that another person is sad, but instead of comforting that person the child may continue doing what they are doing showing little to no disregard for the sad person.

Managing Emotions

When a person gets to the stage where they are able to perceive and understand emotions, as well as use them to facilitate thought, they are then able to manage their own emotions and also able to help others to manage theirs. These people are going to be level headed sorts that are not prone to have emotional outbursts. They will consistently match situations with the proper emotional responses. When they feel that they are getting emotional they will take steps to get control of their emotions.

Chapter 2

Primary Emotional Needs of Children

Body Language

Unlike adults, children use body language to express themselves. Some of the more familiar non-verbal communications of children that you may notice when they are upset are:

they have become withdrawn and are not participating in activities

they have become very quiet and aloof

they may not be responding to you like they usually do

Child Needs

Even though each child is unique and different they still all have the same basic needs. The only difference is in the degree of which each child needs. Some children may want more than others when it comes to attention. Some will demand that you pay attention to their emotional needs or will wait for your attention. The keyword to keep in mind here is moderation.

Give the child what they need but do not over indulge them.

Explain to your child that you love them but that you need to work so that you can provide your family with a good life. Even if it seems like your child does not understand what you are saying to them still take the time to tell them anyway. Eventually, they will begin to understand that you are not just a working machine but a person.

Children's needs will not always stay the same. Depending on what has been going on in your child's life, their needs will vary.

Cultivate your own emotional intelligence so that you are able to notice the varying needs of your child and be ready to offer them the support that they will need.

Emotional Support

When it comes to emotional support, children are immature so they need proper emotional support from you. This does not mean giving into every whim of theirs. That is the easy way out and that, in the long run, is not helping your child.

Giving your child positive attention is certainly important, they should be made to feel that they are an important part of your life.

You need to find a happy balance when it comes to paying attention towards your child as too much is not good nor is too little.

Making your child realize that they are an important part of your life is important, but also make them aware that you have other priorities in your life such as other children, spouse, work, household chores.

Give them your full attention when you are giving them attention.

Do not multitask while you are attending to them. You do not need to spend countless hours together, but make it a quality time when you do.

Taking ten minutes here and there out of your day to spend some one on one time with your child can build a strong bond between you and your child.

Be understanding when your child does things wrong, they are going to make mistakes which are all part of the learning process. Do not get angry if they do something wrong, instead ask your child to think of a better way of doing a particular thing.

Let them try and figure out the answer before you offer it to them.

Allowing them to try and figure things out will help them to become independent thinkers.

Make sure that you let your child know that making mistakes is all part of learning and life in general.

Tell your child that making mistakes is nothing to be ashamed of and make them aware that we all make mistakes.

This will help them to become more tolerant not only of their own mistakes but those of others as well.

As parents, we all love our children, but on those hectic days where we feel we are being pulled in multiple directions we can sometimes forget to let our child know or remind them that we love them.

Keep in mind that a child needs to be shown that they are loved and told.

You can whisper into your child's ear at the school gate that you love them so that other children don't hear.

Bedtime is a good time to cuddle your child and tell them how much you love them, perhaps read them a bedtime story.

For the emotional welfare of a child, it is important that they have a sense of belonging.

A child should be made to feel that they are a valued member of the family and have a sense that home is their safe zone.

They will begin to wander outside of the family home and begin making friends, but it is still important that the child knows that they have a supportive family and a home to come back to when needed.

The kind of bonds that a child develops with their family will affect the rest of the relationships in their life.

Developing EQ

When developing EQ in children, it is important that you are able to differentiate between what they want versus what their needs are. Often parents find that they give in to what the child wants and then find that their child has completely taken over their lives. They mistake their child's wants with their needs. Wants of children are unlimited whereas on the other hand needs are limited. They all need shelter, clothing, and food as basic needs. But do not need a cell phone, TV, or a big fancy house. It is not just our children that chase after the constant wants, but also parents and adults do the same thing by chasing their wants in life. You should first start to make sure that you have all of your child's needs are taken care of then give them one or two of their wants.

It is good for a child to have boundaries, so they know what rules they are expected to follow to stay within those boundaries. Keep some of their activities time bound such as playtime with friends, what time they must get up during the weekdays. Make sure that they go to the washroom, wash, brushes their teeth and comb their hair etc. Be firm with your child with these routines but not rigid.

If your child refuses to follow a rule, talk to them why they need to follow that rule. Then tell them of the consequence if they do not follow the rule. If for example your child is not washing their face or brushing their teeth or combing their hair, take away something they enjoy such as playing video games. Explain that you do not want their teeth to turn bad if they do not brush their teeth so that they will end up wearing false teeth.

Make sure to tell your child the truth about things so that they don't find out from others what the truth is, this will only lead to them thinking that you lied to them. You could show your appreciation to your child for going back to brushing his teeth by spending some quality time with them. Perhaps the two of you could go for a bike ride and stop for a smoothie to enjoy in the park together.

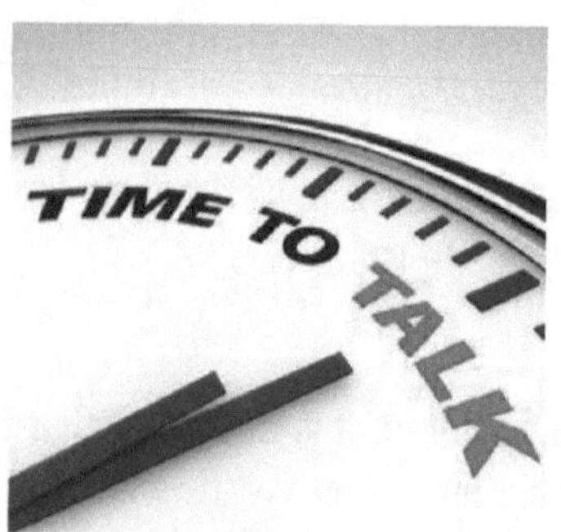

Communication

Having good communication skills so that you are able to interact with your child is very important in helping you to understand your child better. You want your child to sense that they are able to approach you and talk with you about any problems they may be facing. But in order for this to happen you must build up a trusting relationship with your child. If you are the kind of person that spends more time preaching, being overly judgmental and strict, it is less likely that your child will not approach you as they will not feel comfortable in confiding in you. Worse, if they feel scared to approach you. Make sure to maintain a good balance between your being an authoritative figure in your child's life to being a friend. Work at being open and honest with your child.

Explain to your child why it is that you insist that they do certain things in a certain way, also make sure to point out to them that you yourself have made mistakes and when you do with your child, make sure to apologize for the mistakes. Show your child that you are human and do make mistakes. Your child will respect you for this and instead of looking at you as some kind of superhuman they will see you as a person.

Even when you do have good communication with your child it can be hard to try and encourage them to share their feelings with you. With a younger child try asking them the same questions at different times, encouraging them to open up to you. Make sure to ask them how they are feeling. Tell your child that you are both on the same team and that you can share anything with each other. Also tell your child that you will not yell or scream at them for telling you the truth.

Ask your child about their interests, and who their school friends are. These questions will show your child that you are interested in them and what they are doing. Ask them questions throughout the day instead of firing a bunch of questions at them at once. Share some of your childhood stories with them, this can help encourage them to share theirs.

If you sense that your child may be dealing with a bully let him know that he has the right to defend himself. Tell them ways that they can handle the bully. Make sure to follow up with your child to see if they have managed to take care of the bully situation. If on the other hand you find that it is your child that is being a bully, you will need to teach your child how to become more aware of others emotions. You will also need to try and figure out where this behavior stems from. Is your child seeing fights at home? In most cases if you can find the root cause of the bullying behavior often it will help resolve the problem.

Chapter 3

Methods to Use to Teach Emotional Intelligence

The majority of EI formation occurs from birth to the age of 21, building emotional intelligence starts at birth and continues into adulthood. Parents will have the most influence over their child from age 13 and under. By the time a child reaches 13 years of age, their parents EI influence begins to decline. The most productive time is during the ages of 2 to 6 years of age. Children at these stages are able to recognize emotions and develop thinking for themselves. By the time children have reached middle school, it becomes much more difficult for parents to emotionally influence them. At this point in time they begin to separate from their parents and more of their instruction begins to come from peers, which can be very good or very bad, depending on the type of peers they are keeping company with and the situation.

Children are very receptive to emotional coaching during these formative years because they are very detail orientated, socially aware as well as receptive to instruction from parents.

Method 1: Self-development and Modeling

While many of the following methods will involve picking and choosing what is going to work best for you and your child, the first method is a must for everybody involved. Parents are natural models for their children, so it is best to do it intentionally.

You can model for your child by showing your child the appropriate action for any given situation. To make sure it has a good effect try and use an authentic approach. For children acting and reality are largely the same, until about kindergarten age, that is when they begin to draw very sharp contrasts between fantasy and reality. Your school age child will know the difference between acting out something and actually doing it for real. Actually doing it is much more meaningful for them.

Make sure that what you are modeling is authentic. It is hard for you to model a behavior that you as the parent are not familiar with. The best way that you can help in developing your child's emotional intelligence is to improve and develop your own. Examine your emotions when you are interacting with others in front of your child, those that you interact with regularly in front of your child. Such as other family members, teachers, and friends.

Method 2: Actions During Infancy

During infancy is when your child's basic sense of trust and fear is formed, this is when the foundation for high emotional intelligence is made. Follow the steps below to help form high EI during infancy.

1. When an infant cries respond to their cries quickly and appropriately. When a baby's basic social and biological needs are not met, a baby will always cry. You cannot spoil an infant. With a quick response to their cries, this will help to set the psychological foundation for trust.

2. Keep yourself calm around your infant, as they can be very perceptive of picking up on any anxiety you may be feeling. You will keep your baby calm if you stay calm. As your baby develops they will have better emotional control if they have consistently low anxiety. The reverse is also true.

3. Infants view unmet needs as life-threatening conditions, make sure to always soothe your baby. If there is a need of theirs that has not been met they may continue to cry until they are completely exhausted and unable to continue. By soothing your baby, you will help their nervous system to develop, training their nervous system to self-soothe. This final foundation of self-soothing ability will help with the management of emotions later in life.

Method 3: Acknowledge & Identify Emotions

As children learn how to express themselves beyond crying, they are going to be searching for ways to identify feelings. Do not ignore your child's expression of emotions whether it is crying, laughing, arguing, or throwing a tantrum. You cannot coach emotions until your child has learned to identify them. You can tell your child outright that you can see that they are displaying emotions by saying something like "I can see that you are very angry right now," or "isn't it fun to laugh out loud when you are happy?" Your child will begin to create connections with these statements between the two abstractions of emotions and language to help your child with self-expression. Never squash your child's emotions or argue with them about what they are feeling. You should always try to nurture your child's self-expression, this will help them to become readily able to communicate with their expression of feelings.

Method 4: Empathize and Never Repress

Often parents end up damaging their child's emotional intelligence with the best intentions. By telling their child something like "boys don't cry" or "girls should never feel that way" they are guiding their child toward what their idea of a proper emotional display is.

Instead what they may be doing is damaging their child's own emotional security. A child's emotions are real and serious and we should treat them as such at all times. Even if the emotion your child is having does not make sense in your adult brain, always empathize with your child. Don't dismiss their feelings or try to distract from them, but instead embrace and acknowledge them.

Let your child know that it is okay to feel however they feel, because you are instructing emotions and this will not make them go away. A child does not see any difference between their emotions and their sense of self. When you deny a child's emotion, you are basically denying the child's self. Just because you instruct a child to dismiss the emotion this will not stop the emotion, it merely trains your child to repress it, and there is almost nothing more damaging to EI than a habit of repressing emotion.

Method 5: Teach Problem Solving

Managing emotions and problem solving go hand-in-hand. There is always a cause behind emotions. When unwanted emotions flare up, correcting the situation is a problem-solving exercise. Your child needs to learn to develop internal problem solving to manage their emotions, they must also develop external problem solving so that they are able to deal with the emotions of others.

Method 6: Encourage Appropriate Expression

Encouraging appropriate expression goes very well with method four. Often a child will express negative emotion in the most dramatic way or convenient way possible for them to get the reaction they are seeking. They may hit someone or something or engage in other forms of inappropriate behavior. In situations such as these many parents make a mistake. They discipline the child, trying to teach them, that behavior like that is not appropriate. While they are trying to teach their child this, they are also at the same time repressing the emotion that caused the action in the first place. Instead of disciplining your child in the "traditional sense," guide your child towards a correct display of emotion and teach them that it is okay to feel angry, hurt, sad or frustrated. Explain to your child that there are right ways to express emotions. Hitting someone is not a right way to express those emotions. Instead suggest that they try hitting a pillow or going for a run or taking a time out to calm down.

If your child tends to throw and break things when they get angry, try to encourage them to release this pent up energy through crying instead. Try and teach your child that it is okay to cry and release their frustration, especially boys. Let your boy know that it is okay for boys to cry. Explain to them that it is one of the best ways to release any built up emotions they are feeling and they will feel much better after a good cry.

Method 7: Play

Children learn a lot through playing and acting out certain situations either directly or indirectly. When you see a negative pattern of behavior during play step in and turn the negative into an instructional and entertaining game.

Method 8: Emotion Talks- diffuse tension with emotion talk

This is a method that works best with school age children who are capable of talking and carrying on a conversation. When emotions are running especially high this is when an emotion talk can be used. It will diffuse the tension of the situation, reinforce the parent-child relationship, this will help your child to identify the feelings that caused the situation and gives them ideas on how to deal with it in the future.

Method 9: Wish Fulfillment

This is a method to use when your child has inappropriate or impossible desires to fulfill. Research has shown that the brain can feel fulfilled just by imagining the fulfillment of a desire, basically in the same way if the event had actually come true. This goes to show the power of the human imagination.

Repressing or denying desires usually ends up causing conflict that could end up escalating. Coach your child to imagine that their desire was fulfilled. For example, have them imagine that they are eating the banana sundae they wanted just before dinner time, picturing the sweet taste of the nice cold ice cream. This satiety will fade, but it will give you some time to get dinner prepared to replace the imagined banana split.

When the basic needs are met, you can then have an appropriate conversation about the appropriate way to meet needs. In the above example when your child wanted a banana split just before dinner, this is when you explain to your child that it is not appropriate to eat sweet treats right before dinner.

Chapter 4

Ways to Apply Methods in Everyday Fashion

We can talk about methodology until we are blue in the face, but really understanding it and knowing how to put it into place are two very different challenges. All the methods in chapter 3 can be used in slightly different ways, with the exception of method two. In this chapter, we are going to take a look at the everyday actions you as a parent can apply these methods to help develop your child's emotional intelligence.

Applying Method 1: Modeling

To start with you must start to do things every day that are going to improve your own emotional intelligence, to make you an exemplary model for your child. This you must do before you even consider instructing your child.

Keep a Record of Your Emotions: Write a Journal

By keeping a journal, you can keep track and record daily your emotions and what caused them. You will then be able to use this collected data to see your own patterns. Have you noticed a pattern where you tend to lose your emotional composure with a certain person or particular situation?

List Your Triggers: Learn What are your "Hot Buttons"

We all have certain "hot buttons" that will trigger negative reactions from us. Often with parents the source of their "hot buttons" comes from their children. Write a list of all of your hot buttons in your journal that you can think of. Now write down the common reaction you seem to have with each of your "hot buttons." After reviewing your list you may feel a bit embarrassed, but now write down the way that you wish that you had reacted. You want to choose a reaction that is positive or at least constructive and goes well with the other key things in fostering emotional intelligence. You can pick one "hot button" to work on each week and keep practicing your chosen alternate reaction until it eventually becomes a habit.

Talk About Your Goals: Discuss with Your Spouse

You need to keep a boundary between yourself and child but talk with your spouse, close friend or counselor about your goals. You will find that your spouse can offer some great insight into your reactions in different situations.

Their information can help finish your list of "hot button" reactions.

Use Positive Reinforcement: Include Everyone

In this one, you can include everyone, your child included. Make a simple statement to your loved ones stating that you are trying to get better at how you react to certain situations or problems. Show them that you have put a penny jar on the counter, explain to them that every time that you react the right way and do the right thing, a penny will be put into the jar. This is a form of reinforcement that you can use for everyone of appropriate age who is practicing their emotional intelligence. Filling up the penny jar can become a family goal. The rest of the modeling is reminding you to take the appropriate action in different situations that you find yourself in.

Applying Method 3: Response-based Approach

With this method you want to take the opportunity to name an emotion, both positive and negative, jump on the opportunity by simply naming the emotion and the context that you see, but also in a way that feels natural and that your child can make sense of.

The best way to use this method is with consistency. Keep it simple, do not bombard your child with many different words for the one emotion. Pick one word and use that word consistently to express that emotion. For example when you are teaching your child to identify with "angry" do not use other words to express this emotion such as raging, fuming, wild with rage etc. Instead pick one word and stick with it. Use that one word until your child gains understanding by using the word himself.

Some, parents, use tools such as the "mood meter" that visualizes feelings on a spectrum and prompts the child to identify where on the meter they are and where they should be.

Applying Method 4: Always Show Empathy to Your Child

For a healthy emotional development of a child, it is important that as a parent you show your child empathy. Always show empathy even if the emotion is not one that you understand or don't agree with.

1. Take your child and sit them down in a comfortable spot to talk if it is possible.

2. Express to your child what emotion it is that you see with a statement like, "I can see that you are frustrated right now."

3. Show your child that you accept the emotion and more importantly that you are okay with it.

4. Soothe your child and give them reinforcement until they feel better. Don't attempt to invalidate their feelings or distract them from their feelings. If it is appropriate talk to them about why they are having these feelings and what they can do to deal with the situation. This often leads into method 8: the emotion talk.

Applying Method 5: Problem Solving

Learning to problem solve is an important skill for every child to learn. Here are the basics of problem solving. Eventually, children will internalize this but at first you need to supervise the process.

1. Get calmed down

The child may have multiple strategies for this, including leaving the situation, or taking slow breaths, or holding onto a special comfort object.

2. Identify the emotions and the cause

You need to prompt your child to identify a feeling, such as angry or sad. Then ask them to identify the cause of their emotional reaction.

3. Talk about appropriate solutions and rules

If for example there is a recurring problem, prep your child with the steps they can take prior to the situation. This can help a child that may be getting bullied in some way by another child. Perhaps a child keeps drawing on your child's drawing paper in class, this is a form of bullying. Instruct your child to tell the teacher of the other child's inappropriate behavior towards them.

You can give your child multiple appropriate solutions depending on the problem and make sure to encourage them to choose one. They might try to share their feelings with the other child or they may need to get an adult to help them with the situation. Always remind your child to be calm and respectful regardless of the solution they choose.

Applying Method 6: Encourage Expression in Your Child

It is important that you encourage your child to express themselves. If your child is having a temper tantrum then you need to find a way to channel their energy into something else. You can encourage other types of expression with older children such as drawing, or writing, or making music to express themselves. Here are some ideas:

1. Write a letter

Even if this letter is never going to be read by the person it is intended for, simply by getting out what you wish you could say to them is a great way for literate children to express themselves.

2. Rip paper

The ripping of paper is a great way to release emotional tension, it works for preschool children as well. This is a less destructive form of emotional release than the alternative. The child can rip up paper into a waste paper basket until they have calmed down.

3. Act out a skit

You can act out a little play with your child, you can pretend to be the person that they are having trouble with. This will help give your child some emotional release, and a chance to practice proper expression.

4. Compose a song or poem

Your child can write a song, poem or tune that conveys their emotion. They may share it if they wish or they can choose to keep it private—do not force them to share it if they do not wish to.

Applying Method 7: Constructive Play

Constructive play is more like a skit or game the message that you as a parent want to convey to your child. Make sure to make the game fun and unstructured. Do not try and force the message onto your child. Just set up the play or skit scenario and let it take its course. It may not work as you had hoped, but the main thing is that it was fun and your child will probably want to play it again. You may have to repeat the skit many times before the message is internalized by your child.

Applying Method 8: Emotion Talks

One of the most challenging and effective ways to raise your child's emotional intelligence is with emotion talks. These cannot be faked and must be applied to a real situation.

1. Make sure to be calmed down. No one is able to talk constructively when emotions are running high.

2. Find a place that is comfortable and quiet, never make a public display of an emotion. Sit in a calm surrounding and talk with your child. Make this talk something between just the two of you.

3. It is important that you validate all of the emotions that are involved,

including your own, as well as your child's so that everyone involved knows the feelings of each other.

4. Remind your child that you are talking to them not to punish them, but to help them work through their feelings and help solve the problem.

5. Find out what is causing these emotions, and come up with solutions for each cause.

6. Talk to your child about the consequences of not dealing with emotions in the right way.

7. Explain to your child that it is okay for them to feel however they feel, but it is their responsibility to control what they do with those feelings and act appropriately.

8. Always end these discussions with your child with an affirmation that you love them and that you are there to help them. Emotion talks only last a few minutes. They help to deepen the parent-child relationship and touch on all branches of emotional intelligence.

Applying Method 9: Enhancing Your Child's Imagination

You can usually just have your child close their eyes and imagine the possibilities in their head. There are also several things that you can do with your child to enhance their imagination or take a different approach.

1. Act out their desire

If it is appropriate they can act out their desire in a fantasy setting. If your child wants to shoot a paintball gun, but they are still too young, you can encourage them to pretend their plastic gun is a paintball gun. Explain to them when they turn a certain age then they can try the real paintball gun if they wish.

2. Draw or write about their desire

Bring out the art supplies and encourage your child to make a story or draw or paint a picture about their desire. After they have completed their creation you can talk with them about it.

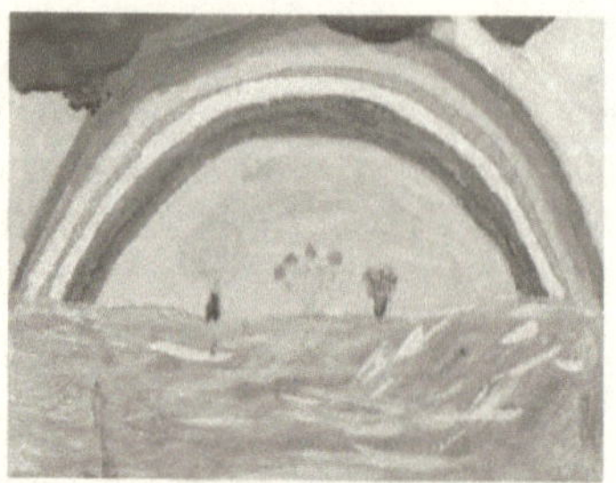

Chapter 5

Giving Your Child an EQ Quiz

Ask your child the questions below to find out what their present emotional intelligence level is. If your child is young and his vocabulary is very limited you will need to explain the meaning of the questions and the answer choices to him in a way that he will understand.

Questions:

1. List five of your friends:

1.

2.

3.

4.

5.

After each of the name, write whether that friend is aggressive, sensitive, or cooperative.

2. When I get upset while playing with other children,

(Tick or mark the correct answer.)

a. I leave them and I come back home

b. I speak to them and let them know what exactly upset me.

c. I shout at them and do not let them play.

d. I talk to an adult like my teacher and complain about that child that is upsetting me.

3. How happy are you with who you are? Would you like to change:

a. Your hair

b. Your height

c. Changes that you are seeing happening with your body (bodily changes, facial hair).

d. None

4. When I make mistakes,

(Tick the right answer)

a. Try and correct my mistake

b. I shout and throw things

c. Think that I am no good

d. Try and hide it from everyone

5. How would you respond to these situations? Would you be comfortable, uncomfortable, or feel like running away.

Please write C for comfortable, U for uncomfortable, and RA for feel like running away, after the question.

a. When you are given a task that is very difficult to do

b. When someone is criticizing you

c. When people are angry

d. When people are crying

6. How often do you fight or have disagreements with others?

a. Never

b. Many times in a month

c. A few times in a month

d. All the time

7. Do you like to talk to new kids of your own age?

a. No

b. Yes

8. How many friends do you have in total at home and school?

a. More than 5

b. Less than 5

c. None

9. I get angry when:

a. Somebody insults or abuses me

b. I do not win

c. Others who do not do what I tell them to do

d. When others isolate me

10. Do you think that you can learn mountain climbing and climb Mount Everest when you grow up?

a. I might

b. Yes

c. No

d. I don't know

Answers

Your child has a high emotional intelligence if he answered the questions as follows:

Q1 Answer: You are the judge!

Q2 Answer: b. Tell them exactly what upset me

Q3 Answer: None

Q4 Answer: c. Try to correct them

Q5 Answer: More than one C's

Q6 Answer: a few times a month

Q7 Answer: a. Yes

Q8 Answer: c. More than five

Q9 Answer: d. Somebody insults or abuses me

Q10 Answer: c. Yes

The four building blocks of emotional intelligence help us to align our emotions and to manage others'. They are the following:

1. Self-awareness

2. Self-management

3. Social-awareness

4. Relationship management

1. Self-awareness

Being aware of how we feel is the first step towards managing our emotions. We can align with the truth of our personality when we have self-awareness. It tells you exactly what you are and are not good at. With your child, as they develop and mature, he will become better at expressing his emotions. To help develop self-awareness in children you need to teach them to think of what they did, teach them to make decisions on their own, as well as spend time on reflecting on things. It is a good idea that you encourage the child to judge their actions as appropriate or inappropriate.

2. Self-management

You can introduce self-management with simple things to your child. Self-management with smaller children can start with putting their toys in their proper places. You can set up certain tasks for them to do in a day. This will help your child to remember things and to do things on time.

3. Social-awareness

Children have their first interactions through adults. Children learn how to act in front of others by watching how you act towards others. Once they start playing with other children, they begin to learn how to manage their emotions better. When they are attending the school they develop their own independent social life apart from their parents.

4. Relationship Management

One of the most important factors for our happiness is relationships with others. It is important that we teach our children the importance of relationships and giving them the ability to manage relationships, this is essential to help ensure that they will develop good relationships as adults. Getting the best results out of a situation is what relationship management is all about.

Teaching your child to be emotionally intelligent is very important for their future happiness and success in life. The more their EQ is developed, it will ensure that they will get on well with others in life. Not only will we develop our children's EQ but inadvertently we will improve our own emotional intelligence.